If You Want What We Have

A Journey Through The Twelve Steps Of Recovery
A Workbook And Guide To The Twelve-Step Process

by Rev. Dr. Kevin T. Coughlin Ph.D.

KTC Publishing Phase IIC Coaching, LLC

This book is a work of nonfiction.

First Printing

Printed in the United States of America

ISBN 978-0-9977006-8-8 (paperback)

Foreword

Author, Dr. Rev. Kevin T. Coughlin Ph.D., DCC, DDVA, DLC, DD, NCIP, NCAMP, IMAC has written an important piece of work with his book release titled; If You Want What We Have: A Journey Through the Twelve Steps of Recovery. An amazing workbook that guides those using a twelve-step program gain insight, wisdom, and sees their growth in recovery while they complete each of the twelve steps. An excellent companion guide and workbook for anyone to get the clearest direction from any addiction to reclaim one's life.

Reverend Coughlin is a Founder and the Director of New Beginning Ministry, Inc., an evidence-based, twelve-step residential addiction recovery program for adults that is accredited by the A.A.C.T. Rev. Coughlin has helped thousands of people to change their lives over the past nineteen plus years. A devout believer in the twelve-step program, he has seen firsthand how it can transform lives, including himself and many family members.

Dr. Kevin Coughlin has written two more books titled; In The Sunlight of the Spirit, and, Addictions: What all Parents Need to Know to Survive the Drug Epidemic. Kevin shares much of his decades of experiences as he too lives life in recovery and shares his vast knowledge and education throughout all his books to help save many lives from the grasp of addiction.

You will find and learn the skills and tools to use as you gain understanding about addiction, the cycle, and behaviors with the many facts and illustrations that will help the reader navigate redemption into sobriety within the pages of this workbook. Well-written, clear format guide that makes working the twelve steps enjoyable and with ease. A must read guide for anyone looking to recover from addiction.

Catherine Townsend-Lyon, Author of Addicted to Dimes, Recovery Columnist for in Recovery Magazine. Catherine Townsend-Lyon is TGK Publishers Best Selling Author with her shocking debut Memoir "Addicted to Dimes, (Confessions of a Liar and a Cheat)," available on Amazon, Barnes and Noble and www.addictedminds.com.

Catherine has fast become well-known in the addiction & recovery communities. Her book shares her raw, unedited and haunting past of gambling addiction and alcohol abuse, living with mental/emotional health challenges, and as a childhood trauma and abuse survivor, she helps many in recovery as she advocates for all these important issues to shatter stigma around those who are 'touched' by the same, and sharing HOPE to others in recovery.

Catherine has been invited and featured on many 'Internet Radio shows' as guest author, has been interviewed and written about in a major media article release by, Columbia University titled, "Gambling with America's Health".

If you want what we have; a journey through the twelve steps of recovery workbook and manual has been used successfully by numerous individuals, residential recovery programs, out-patient programs, professional recovery coaches, aftercare professionals, counselors, therapists, probation officers, ministries, recovery retreats, sponsors, sober companions, and family members.

Please visit www.theaddiction.expert for more publications written by Rev. Kev. coming soon, and for all of your recovery needs.

Table of Contents

Rev. Dr. Kev's Social Media Accounts

Introduction

When I was seven years old, I accompanied my mother to many twelve-step meetings and witnessed the miracle as it changed her life and mine. A few decades later, the twelve steps saved my life, my brother's life, his wife's life, my uncle's life, and countless friend's lives. After witnessing the power of the twelve-step process my family, friends, and I opened a twelve-step recovery program and retreat in The Poconos of Pennsylvania for adult men and women who suffer from addiction, over the past two decades the thousands of miracles that I have witnessed, and lives saved are due to the twelve-step process.

I felt it was my obligation to share what I have learned over the past forty-seven years about addiction recovery and the twelve-step process. I originally got clean and sober at a twelve-step retreat that was started by one of the Founders of Alcoholics Anonymous, Bill W., it was at this retreat that I started to realize that I had a calling on my life to help other sick and suffering alcoholics and substance abusers.

After two decades of teaching on addiction recovery and the twelve-step process, and developing my skills as a professional writer, it only made sense to combine the two and share this life-saving information with a larger audience. My mom passed on five years ago with over forty years of sobriety, and today I celebrate nineteen years!

My dream is to share my knowledge with as many individuals as I can during my lifetime, building an army of twelve-step professionals who can help save lives. It doesn't matter if you are reading this book for yourself, a family member, or a dear friend; the information contained within the pages here can be life changing. I know that these steps changed and saved my life!

*"It works if you work it, so work it, you're worth it***!" Anonymous**

They say in the rooms of recovery, if you want what we have, and are willing to go to any length to get it, you will recover. All you have to do is want it, and do the footwork. This amazing workbook/manual will aid you on your journey. My personal website is www.revkevsrecoveryworld.com I hope you will visit. Best of life!

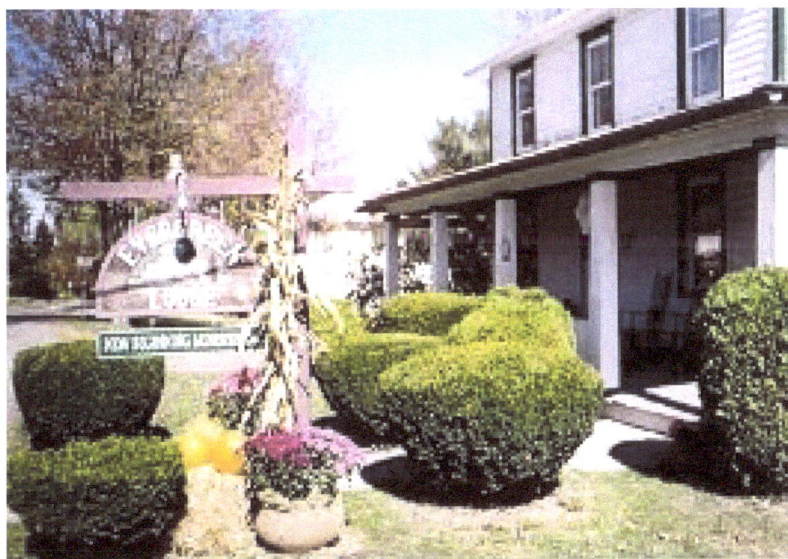

Definitions

Addiction: The repetition of a behavior despite the negative consequences or a neurological impairment leading to such behaviors. Addictions can include, but are not limited to, substance abuse, process addictions: exercise addiction, food addiction, computer addiction, and gambling. Classic signs of addiction include impaired control over substances or behavior, obsession with substance or behavior, continued use despite negative consequences and denial. Habits and patterns associated with addiction are usually characterized by immediate gratification, coupled with delayed harmful effects.

Physiological dependence can occur when the body has to adjust to the substance by combining the substance into its "normal" functioning. This state creates the conditions of tolerance and withdrawal. Withdrawal refers to physical and psychological symptoms when reducing or discontinuing a substance that the body has become dependent upon.

Withdrawal: Is the body's reaction to abstaining from a substance of which it has become dependent. Without the substance, physiological functions that were dependent on the substance will react because of the body's tolerance and dependence on the substance.

Relapse: In relation to drug or alcohol misuse, is resuming the use of a drug or a chemical substance after one or more periods of abstinence.

Alcoholism: Alcohol is the most commonly used substance in the nation, 17.6 million people, or one in every twelve adults—8%, suffer from alcohol abuse or dependence along with several million more who engage in risky drinking behaviors that could lead to alcoholism or problem drinking.

More than half of all adults have a family history of alcoholism or problem drinking, and more than seven million children live in a household where at least one parent is alcohol dependent or has abused alcohol.

Drug Dependence: According to the National Survey on Drug Use and Health (NSDUH), an estimated 20 million Americans aged twelve or older have used an illegal drug in the past month. This estimate represents 8% percent of the population older than age twelve. Nonmedical use or abuse of prescription drugs such as painkillers, sedatives, and stimulants is growing, with an estimated forty-eight million people ages twelve and older using prescription drugs for nonmedical reasons. This affects approximately twenty percent of the US population.

Alcoholism and drug dependence can affect all aspects of a person's life, including serious health complications affecting virtually every organ in the body and the brain; it can also damage emotional stability, finances, career, and impact family, friends and the entire community in which an alcoholic or drug abuser lives.

Powerlessness: Can't use-physical allergy (phenomenon of craving); Can't quit-mental obsession; Can't change on our own power, on will power (self-will); Can't control—unmanageability; Can't trust-no-one nor any being is going to help us protect us, support us.

Sanity/Insanity: Sanity—Completeness/wholeness of mind, the ability to see the truth.

Insanity—Lack of wholeness of mind, inability to see the truth; doing the same thing over and over, and expecting a different result. Insanity doesn't mean we are "crazy;" we lack the knowledge (agnostic) and are unable, to see the truth. It becomes hard to differentiate between the truth and the false.

Belief: Taking the Word of others and acting upon it, putting their suggestions into practice (Le. -we believe and trust the word(s) of the first 100 in AA as spelled out in the ***BB-Alcoholics Anonymous***). *"Belief means reliance, not defiance"*-Page 31, the ***12 & 12***. It's okay to rely on someone with more experience, strength, and hope than us. If we are doubtful or suspicious, it shows us that we still have too healthy an Ego that is all too eager to run the show. What we believe shows. If we are consistently cheerful, positive and optimistic, it shows we believe things are going to turn out all right. If we are consistently down, glum, grouchy, pessimistic and negative, we show that we expect the worst is going to happen; we are operating out of self-will (fear, distrust, suspicion, doubt).

Faith: Is the substance (it materializes) of things hoped for, the evidence of things not seen. It is not seeing but believing. The best example I can give. Which is also stated in the BB, is that one month, two months, three months or six months down the road, I can see dramatic changes/ transformations in people that work the program of action—the Steps; they might not even see it. But I do! All that is asked in this program. Initially, is "believe what we believe, and you will develop your belief in the Higher Power/God of your understanding". Some of the characteristics of faith are- we stop struggling, we stop trying to make things happen, we let go and let God-all of this can be summed up in one word-humility.

Humility: *"Is a clear recognition of what and who we are. Followed by a sincere attempt (action-steps) to become (change/transformation) what we could be."* Page 58, ***12 & 12***. *"God does for me what I could not do for myself."* Some terms that describe humility are-risk, vulnerable, leap of faith, God in charge, right proportioned, truthful, honest, seeking and doing my Higher Power will.

Relapse Prevention: Attempts to group the factors that contribute to relapse into two broad categories: immediate determinants and covert antecedents.

Immediate determinants are the environmental and emotional situations that are associated with relapse, including high-risk situations that threaten an individual's sense of control, coping strategies, and outcome expectancies. Covert antecedents, which are less obvious factors influencing relapse, include lifestyle factors such as stress level and balance, and urges and cravings. The relapse prevention model teaches substance abusers to anticipate relapse by recognizing and coping with various immediate determinants and covert antecedents. The RP model shows the greatest success with treatment of alcoholism, but it has not been shown to be superior to other treatment options.

A Twelve-Step Program: Is a set of guiding principles (sometimes accepted by members as being 'spiritual principles') outlining a course of action for tackling problems including alcoholism, drug addiction, and compulsion.

Originally proposed by Alcoholics Anonymous (AA) as a method of recovery from alcoholism, the original Twelve Steps were first published in the 1939 book ***Alcoholics Anonymous***: The Story of How More Than One Hundred Men Have Recovered from Alcoholism. The method was adapted and became the foundation of other twelve-step programs.

As summarized by the American Psychological Association, the initial twelve steps involved the following:

• Admitting that one cannot control one's alcoholism, addiction, or compulsion
• Recognizing a higher power that can restore sanity
• Examining past errors with the help of a sponsor (experienced member)
• Making amends for these errors
• Learning to live a new life with a new code of behavior
• Helping others who suffer from the same alcoholism, addictions or compulsions.

The Diagnostic and Statistical Manual of Mental Disorders, Fifth Edition, commonly referred to as the ***DSM-V*** or ***DSM 5***, is the latest version of the American Psychiatric Association's gold standard text on the names, symptoms, and diagnostic features of every recognized mental illness, including addictions. This edition was published in May 2013, nearly 20 years after the original publication of the previous edition, the ***DSM-IV***, in 1994.

• Substance Abuse
• Addiction Treatment
• Alcohol Treatment
• Alcohol Abuse
• Opiate Addiction

The ***DSM-V*** recognizes substance-related disorders resulting from the use of ten separate classes of drugs: alcohol, caffeine, cannabis, hallucinogens (phencyclidine or similarly acting arylcyclohexylamines), other hallucinogens such as LSD, inhalants, opioids, sedatives, hypnotics, anxiolytics, stimulants (including amphetamine-type substances, cocaine, and other stimulants), tobacco, and other or unknown substances. Therefore, while some major grouping of psychoactive substances is specifically identified, use of other or unknown substances can also form the basis of a substance related or addictive disorder.

The ***DSM 5*** explains that activation of the brain's reward system is central to problems arising from drug use—the rewarding feeling that people experience as a result of taking drugs may be so profound that they neglect other normal activities in favor of taking the drug. While the pharmacological mechanisms for each class of drug are different, the activation of the reward system is similar across substances in producing feelings of pleasure or euphoria, which is often referred to as a "high".

The ***DSM 5*** also recognizes that people are not all automatically or equally vulnerable to developing substance-related disorders and that some individuals have lower levels of self-control, which may be brain-based, which predispose them to develop problems if exposed to drugs.

There are two groups of substance-related disorders: substance use disorders and substance-induced disorders. Substance use disorders are patterns of symptoms resulting from the use of a substance that the individual continues to take, despite experiencing problems as a result. Substance-induced disorders include intoxication, withdrawal, substance-induced mental disorders, including substance-induced psychosis, substance-induced bipolar and related disorders, substance-induced depressive disorders, substance-induced anxiety disorders, substance induced obsessive-compulsive and related disorders, substance-induced sleep disorders, substance induced sexual dysfunctions, substance-induced delirium, and substance-induced neurocognitive disorders.

Substance use disorders span a wide variety of problems arising from substance use, and cover 11 different criteria:

1. Taking the substance in larger amounts or for longer than the you meant to
2. Wanting to cut down or stop using the substance but not managing to
3. Spending a lot of time getting, using, or recovering from use of the substance
4. Cravings and urges to use the substance
5. Not managing to do what you should at work, home or school, because of substance use
6. Continuing to use, even when it causes problems in relationships
7. Giving up important social, occupational or recreational activities because of substance use
8. Using substances again and again, even when it puts you in danger
9. Continuing to use, even when the you know you have a physical or psychological problem that could have been caused or made worse by the substance
10. Needing more of the substance to get the effect you want (tolerance)
11. Development of withdrawal symptoms, which can be relieved by taking more of the substance.

The *DSM 5* allows clinicians to specify how severe the substance use disorder is, depending on how many symptoms are identified. Two or three symptoms indicate a mild substance use disorder, four or five symptoms indicate a moderate substance use disorder, and six or more symptoms indicate a severe substance use disorder. Clinicians can also add "in early remission," "in sustained remission," "on maintenance therapy," and "in a controlled environment."

* (Information gathered from Wikipedia & AA Literature and other Twelve-Step Programs.)

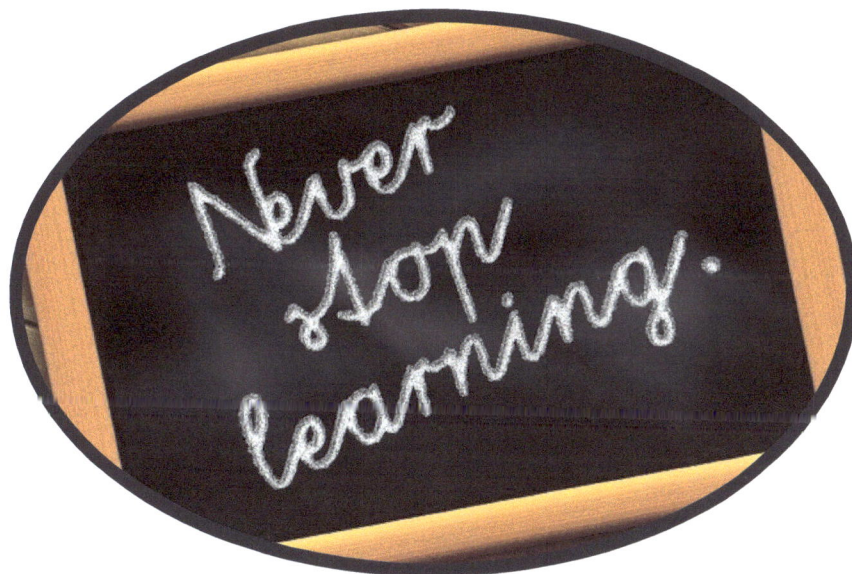

Cultural Perceptions/History

Cultural Perceptions of Addiction and Alcoholism

- In the religious community = sin/ personal trial
- Spiritual = searching for meaning
- Psychological = it's a choice/ symptomatic of underlying condition
- Criminal justice = immoral/ reform
- Medical community = disease/ medically fixable/ chronic
- Socio/cultural = caused by environment/trauma/oppression

Community, Recovery, Treatment

- Modern addiction treatment 1960-1970s
- Staffed largely from local communities of recovery
- Communication between treatment and recovery community
- Professionalization/commercialization the 1980s
- Treatment prices skyrocket
- The spirit of recovery started to shift
- From problem to solution focused
- Recovery community not trusted/ respected by professional community
- Lack of financial support for long-term aftercare
- Evidence-based recovery support protocol
- Lack of peer ethical codes/guidelines
- Weak infrastructures in treatment
- Treatment and recovery community relationship
- Re-criminalization of alcohol and drug problems 80s and 90s leads to new recovery advocacy movement led by faces and voices of recovery and NCADD and local groups.
- The key to future success is unity, teamwork, and communication. Working together for long-term care that is tried, tested, and proven to work. The recovery and treatment community working together to solve this deadly problem.

About Recovery

- There are many different pathways to recovery
- Recovery is self-directed and empowering
- Recovery involves a personal recognition of the need for change
- The root of addiction is self-centeredness, shame is at the core
- Recovery is holistic
- Recovery has many cultural dimensions
- Recovery exists on a continuum of improvement in wellness and overall health
- Recovery is born of gratitude and hope
- Recovery is a process of self-discovery and healing
- Recovery has several support systems
- Recovery involves a process of rebuilding and re-establishing a life and community
- Recovery is a fact!

Problematic News for Treatment

- In the 1950s, the trend toward medicalization and professionalization of treatment started.
- The expansion of Medicaid coverage and private insurance led to physicians, nurses, psychologists, social worker, and other professionals playing a greater role in the treatment field.
- Alcohol and Drug Treatment Systems were separated.
- They merged in the 1990s for one single counselor certification standard.
- Historically addiction treatment has been treated differently than other health problems.
- The Treatment field became very problem focused rather than solution focused.
- Resources for post-treatment became very limited.
- Resources that could have been offered instead of treatment became virtually non-existent.

A Change in Thinking

- Starting in the 1980s a new Recovery Movement Started.
- Increasing stigma associated with growing public support for criminalization of addiction.
- Movement away from medical and public health perspectives.
- 1980s-1990s mandatory sentencing guidelines, 3 strikes you're out!
- SAMHSA established the recovery community support program in 1998.
- 2010 The group FAVOR Faces and Voices in Long-Term Recovery is started to speak as one voice to affect public policy and demonstrate that recovery is working for millions!
- 2015 Research has shown that long-term recovery is most effective.

People/Social/Physical Resources

Recovery Resources Can be Divided Into Three Categories:

A. People Resources: professional recovery coaches, family recovery coaches, case managers, anger management practitioners, gambling addiction coaches, sex addiction coaches, sober companions, prevention professionals, sponsors, recovering peers, clergy, counselors, therapists, doctors, nurses, professors/teachers, social workers, other coaches and professionals, friends, parole and probation, judges, lawyers, law enforcement.

B. Social Resources: recovery meetings, church meetings, Bible studies, sober clubs, sober dances, sober events, employers, colleges/schools, teachers, students, family, friends, co-workers, recovery conventions, webinars, sober parties, sober coffee shops.

C. Physical Resources: sober houses, ¾ houses, community centers, community organizations, employment centers, reliable transportation, financial assistance from family and friends, food, clothing, work clothing, income, benefits, donated items, gas money, rides to meetings.

One important saying in recovery is, ***"You are not alone!"*** it's important that those suffering from addiction realize that there are other people like them, and plenty of people resources to help them to recover.

- Is recovery the priority?
- Only associate with positive people
- Take care of yourself: body, mind, and spirit
- Be true to yourself and recovery
- Experience, strength, and hope outweigh opinions
- Don't put unrealistic expectations on others
- Do you learn by your mistakes?
- It's we, not them!
- Live for today
- Tell the facts; don't lie
- Keep all commitments
- When we give, we get back
- Celebrate even the small victories
- Let your story speak for itself

The Original Twelve Steps

These are the original Twelve Steps as published by Alcoholics Anonymous

1. We admitted we were powerless over alcohol - that our lives had become unmanageable.
2. Came to believe that a Power greater than ourselves could restore us to sanity.
3. Made a decision to turn our will and our lives over to the care of God as we understood Him.
4. Made a searching and fearless moral inventory of ourselves.
5. Admitted to God, to ourselves, and to another human being the exact nature of our wrongs.
6. Were entirely ready to have God remove all these defects of character.
7. Humbly asked Him to remove our shortcomings.
8. Made a list of all persons we had harmed, and became willing to make amends to them all.
9. Made direct amends to such people wherever possible, except when to do so would injure them or others.
10. Continued to take personal inventory, and when we were wrong, promptly admitted it.
11. Sought through prayer and meditation to improve our conscious contact with God as we understood Him, praying only for knowledge of His will for us and the power to carry that out.
12. Having had a spiritual awakening as the result of these steps, we tried to carry this message to alcoholics and to practice these principles in all our affairs.

The Twelve Steps Broken Down Into Simple Form:

Step 1: Gives us the problem	Step 7: Action Step
Step 2: Gives us the solution	Step 8: Action Step
Step 3: A decision to live in the solution	Step 9: Action Step
Step 4: Action Step	Step 10: Growth & Maintenance Step
Step 5: Action Step	Step 11: Growth & Maintenance Step
Step 6: Action Step	Step 12: Growth & Maintenance Step

What Is Addiction?

There are many thoughts on what the problem of addiction is. There are also many opinions on what the solution to addiction is. There are many modalities to choose from. There are so many theories by many different types of people. There is the medical community, the doctors, the clinicians, and the scientists, there is the faith-based community of the Reverends, Rabbis, Yogis, and healers, there are the twelve-step community and grassroots programs. Some addicts rely on self-help. There is Harm Reduction, Emotional Intelligence, Cognitive Behavioral Therapy, Neuroscience, Motivational Interviewing, Inpatient, Outpatient, Aftercare, Medication Assisted Treatment, Detox, Recovery Coaching, Family Recovery Coaching, Interventions, Sober Companions, Sponsors, Peer Mentors, Therapy, Counseling, Sober Housing, Retreats, and twelve-step meetings, and Smart Recovery.

1. In 1934, William D. Silkworth M.D. attended a patient who was alcoholic. Dr. Silkworth said, "I had come to regard him as hopeless." Dr. Silkworth wrote the chapter in "***The Big Book***"
of Alcoholics Anonymous known as *"The Doctor's Opinion."* In this chapter, the doctor describes alcoholism as a disease of the mind, the mental obsession, and a disease of the body, the phenomenon of craving or allergy, or allergy defined is an abnormal reaction.
2. In 1956, The American Medical Association had declared that alcoholism was an illness.
3. In 1991, The AMA further endorsed the dual classification of alcoholism by the International Classification of Diseases under both psychiatric and medical sections.
4. In 2004, The World Health Organization stated that alcoholism is a brain disorder.
5. The American Society of Addiction Medicine and the AMA both maintain that alcoholism is a disease.
6. NAADAC, The Association for Addiction Professionals, believes that Science has shown that addiction is a brain disease that responds well to treatment.
7. The Recovery Community, those in long-term recovery believe that alcoholism is a disease as described by Dr. Silkworth.
8. The Faith-based community is divided some believe that alcoholism is a disease; some believe it's a sin. Different treatment models teach different programs based on what they believe. Some let the client choose what modality they will follow. It's a mixed bag.
9. Most clinicians believe that addiction is a brain disorder.
10. The ASAM defines addiction: as a "primary, chronic disease of the brain with characteristic biological, psychological, social and spiritual manifestations."
11. There are some who feel that addiction comes from an attachment disorder in early childhood or other forms or trauma.

"The man takes a drink or drug, the drink takes a drink (The drug takes a drug), the drink or drug takes the man!"

Logically

Think about this logically for a moment. We are certainly dealing with life and death, so every decision is very important. Let's say you were going to a place that you had never been, a very dangerous place! For our purposes here, we will say that you are on a reality TV show, and you have to spend the weekend in the Everglades in Florida. Let me ask you a question: Would you rather go for the weekend with a guide that had read a book about the Everglades and had some theories, or would you rather go with a guide that had been there many times and made it back alive and was a tried, tested, and proven guide? I think the correct answer is clear.

The recovery community looks at drugs and alcohol as a symptom of the problem, not the problem. If you take the alcohol away from an alcoholic, they still have all of the isms. They will still have the living and the thinking problem that needs to change. They will need a vehicle to change and a support system to support that vehicle. No magic pill is ever going to work as the answer to addiction. The problem defines the solution. If you understand the problem, then you can find a solution to anything. The root cause needs to be dealt with, and the core of addiction, then the symptoms will go away on their own.

We're talking about self-centeredness and shame here as the root and the core of addiction. Living a spirit-centered life will deal with both of these issues. The alcoholic or addict will need the vehicle to go from harmful self or self-centered to spirit-centered. They will also need support for that vehicle to change. A way to identify and understand the problem that they have, so that they can admit and accept that they have it. A solution to solve the problem and a decision that they want to solve it.

They will need an action plan or roadmap to get there, and a plan to maintain their freedom so that they can continue to grow in spirituality.

"I can't, He can; I think I'll let Him!"

Diagrams Of Addiction

A normal person

The spirit will be at the center of the being; everything will be in balance and harmony. The person will function normally without abnormal fears, anger, or harms. The basic instincts will all be in balance as the person continues to grow emotionally and interpersonally.

This diagram represents a person suffering from addiction:

Because the spirit is blocked by self-centeredness or harmful-self, the person cannot grow spiritually, emotionally, or interpersonally. The basic instincts become out of balance such as social, sexual, and security. This causes fears, resentments and harms to others, as well as sexual harms.

13

The basic instincts are now out of balance because of addiction:

The basic instincts will remain out of balance as long as the addicted person's spirit is blocked by harmful-self or self-centeredness. The answer is to live a spirit-centered life based on spiritual principles. The person will need a vehicle to change and a fellowship that supports the change.

The results of addiction:

The result of the basic instincts being out of balance is what you see here. The only way to get rid of these serious life problems is to get back into balance by living a spirit-centered life of sobriety.

Normal people have trouble understanding the mental obsession part of addiction. The phenomenon of craving is easy to understand. a normal person would have to say, why would someone do the same thing over and over again, get into jackpots, and expect different results? that's insanity!

Twelve-Step Programs Are Based On:

1. Principles not personalities
2. Spirituality not religion
3. Progress not perfection
4. Attraction not promotion
5. Honesty not dishonesty
6. Commitment not half measures
7. One day at a time not a race
8. Higher power not your will
9. Program as a vehicle to change you, not you to change program
10. The fellowship supports the program of change, the change doesn't come from the fellowship
11. It's a spiritual program of action, not a selfish program of lazy
12. The twelve-step program works, if you work the twelve-step program.

"MEETING MAKERS MAKE IT IF THEY WORK IT!"

1. Essentially alcoholics and drug addicts use alcohol and drugs because they like the effects produced by drugs and alcohol.
2. After a time, it becomes very difficult for them to differentiate the true from the false.
3. To them, the high life seems like the only normal one.
4. They become restless, irritable, and discontented unless they can again experience the sense of ease and comfort that comes instantly with using their drug of choice.
5. The addict starts with the obsession centered in the mind and finally succumb to the desire again after the phenomenon of craving develops; they pass through the stages of a spree.
6. They emerge remorseful reciting the addict's and alcoholic's National Anthem, "I Promise I Will Never Do That Again!"
7. Unless the addicted person can experience an entire psychic change, there is little hope for them. They much change the way that they live and the way that they think.
8. This behavior will be repeated over and over again unless the entire psychic change takes place.
9. The Moderate drinker has little or no trouble stopping using drugs or drinking if they have a good reason.
10. There is a certain type of addict and alcoholic that uses heavy enough to cause health problems and impair them mentally. It may cause early death or health problems. Sometimes a major change in life structure will lead the person to quit. Falling in love, Doctor warning, environment change, Ill health. Although difficult and troublesome they can stop using.
11. Helping others and service work is the foundation stone of recovery.
12. The Real Addict/Alcoholic at some stage of their using they lose all control, they lose the power of choice and cannot stop. They are without defense against the first drink or drug.
13. Cunning, Baffling, and Powerful, addiction is also progressive and insidious!
14. A spiritual experience may be the only answer to conquering addiction.
15. This is not a comprehensive picture of the true addict/alcoholic, as behavior patterns vary.

Before starting a twelve-step program, an addicted person may need to go to a detox unit to be detoxified from the chemicals they have been using by medical professionals. They may also need to go to a residential addiction recovery facility to get a solid foundation to build their new sober life upon. If the addicted person isn't interested in recovery, an interventionist may be needed to help the family to get their loved one into treatment for their addiction.

The Tools

Tools Needed:

1. AA or NA Basic Text
2. Sponsor AA, NA
3. Personal Daily Journal
4. Anger Log
5. Daily Meditation Books such as "Reflections" or "One Day at a Time."
6. Bible or Recovery Bible (Optional)
7. Twelve and Twelve AA step Book
8. AA or NA Meeting Guide Book
9. Professional Recovery Coach and Case Manager (Optional)
10. Home Group AA NA
11. Address Book to collect Group Member Names & Numbers
12. Professionals to address problems outside the scope of twelve-step programs (If Needed)
13. A specific action plan with goals and objectives, actions to be taken, timetables and follow up.

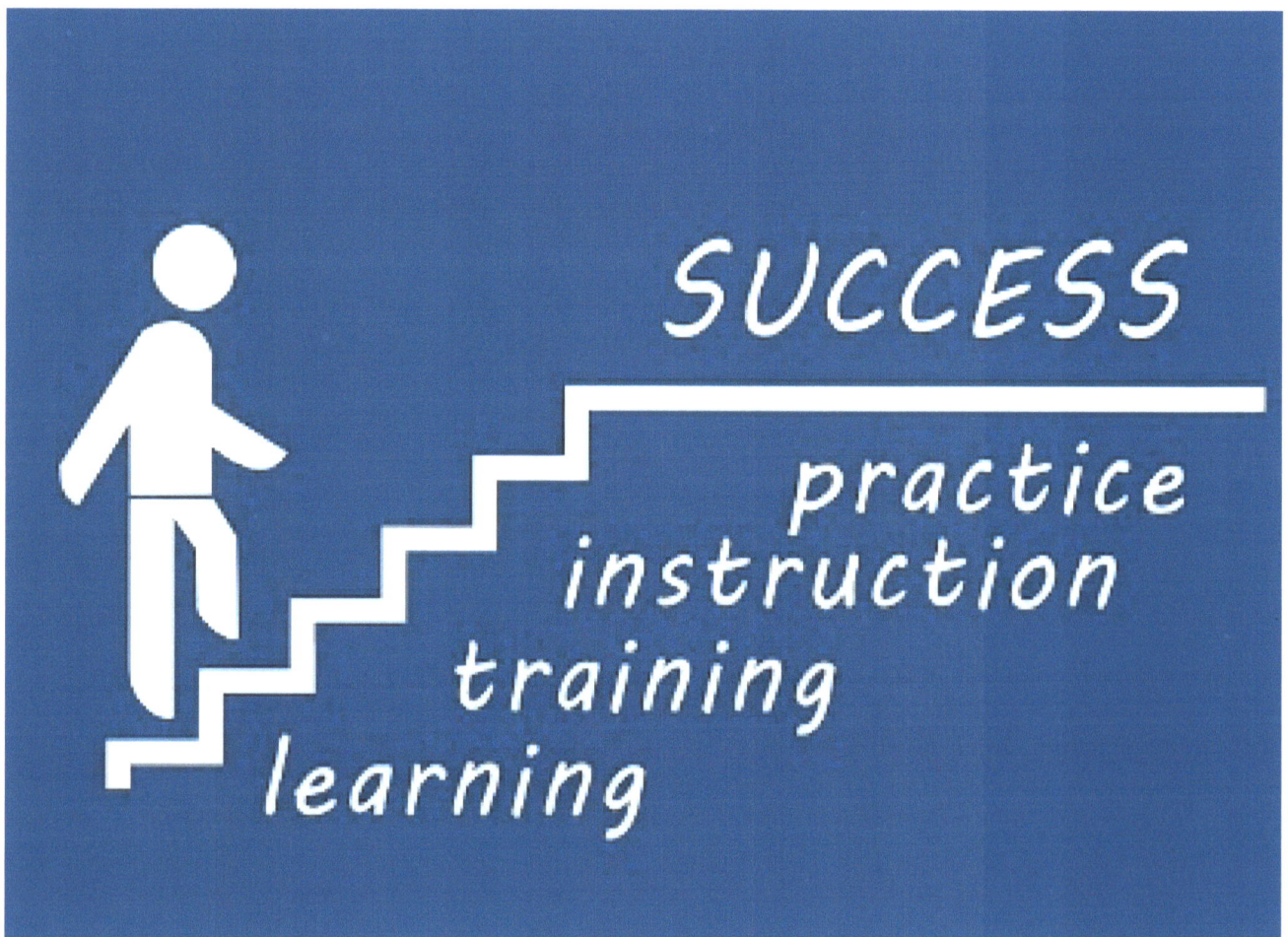

Step One

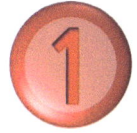

We admitted we were powerless over alcohol - that our lives had become unmanageable.

Step one gives us the problem. For anyone to be able to solve a problem, they have to know what the problem is first. The alcoholic or addict needs to accept and admit that they suffer from addiction. They will need to learn what addiction is so that they can identify. If their drug of choice is alcohol, then they need to learn about the disease of alcoholism. If their drug of choice is opiates, then they need to learn about the disease of addiction. Then they need to be willing to do something about their disease and then take action.

All steps should be worked with a sponsor = A guide to the steps.

Step one requires an admission that the person's life has become unmanageable.

The person needs to hit a bottom, or the bottom needs to be aided by intervention.

There must be consequences for actions without enabling by loved ones and friends.

The person needs to be honest, open-minded, and willing.

When a person hits a bottom, they get uncomfortable in their own skin. They have a moment of clarity where they can see the truth about their life and what they have become. At this point, they may be willing to get help. This window of opportunity is usually short-lived, as the window slams shut rather quickly quite often. Family and friends must act quickly while the window is still open to get their loved one help with their addiction problem.

There is a major difference in the thinking of the recovery community and the scientific community, and the religious community:

A. Scientific Community: Addiction is a brain disorder.

B. Recovery Community: Addiction is a disease of the mind and the body and a spiritual malady.

C. The Religious Community: Addiction is sin and a result of sin.

The Problem defines the solution. It's very important to understand the problem if you want to reach the proper solution, a solution that will work.

Surrender is essential for those that want to recover from this disease. Read the chapter in *The Basic Text* of AA called "The Doctor's Opinion." You will also want to read "Bill's Story" from *The Basic Text*, or *"Big Book."*

1. Think about the price you and your family and friends have paid because of your alcohol and illicit drug use. In the box below list every cost you can think of:

2. In what ways did your life become unmanageable because of your alcohol and illicit drug use? In the box below list all the ways you can think of:

3. Think of all the people who have been hurt and relationships lost because of your addiction. List them in the box below:

4. Please list all the missed opportunities that happened because of your addiction.

5. List the ways you could do damage to your body by using illicit drugs and alcohol.

6. How many times have you blacked out because of illicit drug and alcohol use?_____

7. How many times can you not remember how you got home the night before because of using?_____

8. How many times have you been sick the next day because of using?_____

9. Have you ever isolated from friends and family because of drug and alcohol use? Y/N

10. Have you ever had anger problems because of your drug and alcohol use? Y/N

11. Describe a situation that happened where you felt embarrassed that was related to your illicit drug and alcohol use.

_____
_____.

12. Have you ever felt guilt, remorse, or shame as a result of your using? Y/N

13. Have you made attempts to control your addictive behaviors? Y/N

14. What conclusion have you drawn from your attempts to control your addictive behaviors?

_____.

15. Do you believe that you are powerless over these addictive behaviors? Y/N

16. Have you found yourself in the middle of any jackpots because of using? Y/N

17. If yes, please list jackpots below.

18. Do you ever lie about or hide your using from family or friends? Y/N

19. Do you avoid any family or friends because they don't like your using or behavior when you use? Y/N

20. Can you remember your first drink or drug and how you felt? Y/N

21. If yes, please describe the feeling: _____.

22. Can you remember a time in your life when things started to become unmanageable? Y/N

23. If yes, please describe that period: _____.

_____
_____.

24. Is there an incident or a consequence that happened in your life as a result of using that made you realize that your life was out of control? Y/N

25. How would you conclude that powerlessness and unmanageability play roles in your life as they relate to your addiction:

_____
_____.

26. What are your final conclusions on addiction?

_____
_____.

27. Do you admit and accept that you have a problem and that your life has become unmanageable because of illicit drug use and/or alcohol use? Y/N

28. Are you sure? Y/N

29. Without any reservations? Y/N

30. If your answers are yes, then we can move on to the solution.

If not, talk to your Recovery Coach or Sponsor.

Does this sound about right?

- **Powerless over illicit drugs & alcohol = once started using sooner or later lost control, couldn't control the amount or limit the amount used.**
- **When using illicit drugs and alcohol could not control the negative consequences, that happened as a result of using.**
- **Because of the usage of illicit drugs and alcohol some aspect of life became unacceptable.**

What makes you think that you can no longer use safely?

_____

_____.

What is the difference between admitting and accepting that you have a problem?

_____

_____.

Please list ten reasons why you think that you suffer from addiction or alcoholism.

    1. _____

    2. _____

    3. _____

    4. _____

    5. _____

    6. _____

    7. _____

    8. _____

    9. _____

  10. _____

Step Two

Came to believe that a Power greater than ourselves could restore us to sanity.

Step two gives us the solution to addiction. The problem defines the solution. In step one, we find that the real problem is a lack of power, so the solution must be power. Many people think that this is a religious program; however, it is not. This is a spiritual program based upon spiritual principles. What's important is that the addicted person find a Higher Power, something greater than themselves. A good example of this would be the group as a whole. It could also be Good Orderly Direction. It, of course, can be God if you choose. It's up to each individual to find an "HP" of their understanding.

Please list examples of Higher Powers in the box below:

GOD			
Good Orderly Direction			
Supreme Being			
Power			

Please list examples of what a Higher Power is not in the box below:

A Person			
Coffee Cup			
Self			
Dog			

Remember that it's a Higher Power of your understanding, that you can plug into! Read "There is a Solution" in The Basic Text of AA, and "More About Alcoholism." You will also want to read "We Agnostics."

• Are you willing to lay aside any prejudice you may have? Y/N

• Do you have the willingness to believe in a Power greater than self? Y/N

• Have you come up with your own concept of a Higher Power? Y/N

• Do you admit the possible existence of a Higher Power? Y/N

• Are you honestly willing to seek a Higher Power? Y/N

If you have answered yes to the above five questions, you are on your way to building an effective spiritual structure or foundation of recovery.

Shame is the core of addiction, don't give shame power; there is no shame in being in recovery from addiction!

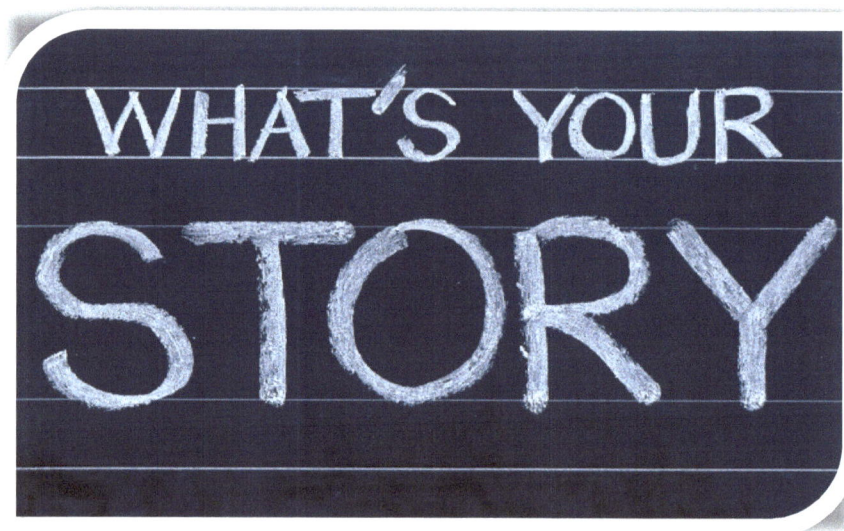

The Basic Text of AA says that we need to have a "*Spiritual Experience*" in order to recover from this disease. This does not mean that you must have a "*mountaintop experience,*" in fact, the majority will not. The Spiritual Experience is about a "*God-Consciousness*" and change.

• Honesty, open-mindedness, and willingness are keys to success in recovery.
• *"Recovery is a daily reprieve contingent upon the maintenance of our spiritual condition."*
• Those who are struggling with turning their lives over to the care of a Higher Power need to look at the fact that every time that they used illicit drugs and alcohol, they turned their lives over to addiction.

Where do you see yourself in five years if you continue to use?

_____
_____.

You have identified the problem of the disease of addiction in step one and the solution to addiction in step two. Next is a decision to be made about the future.

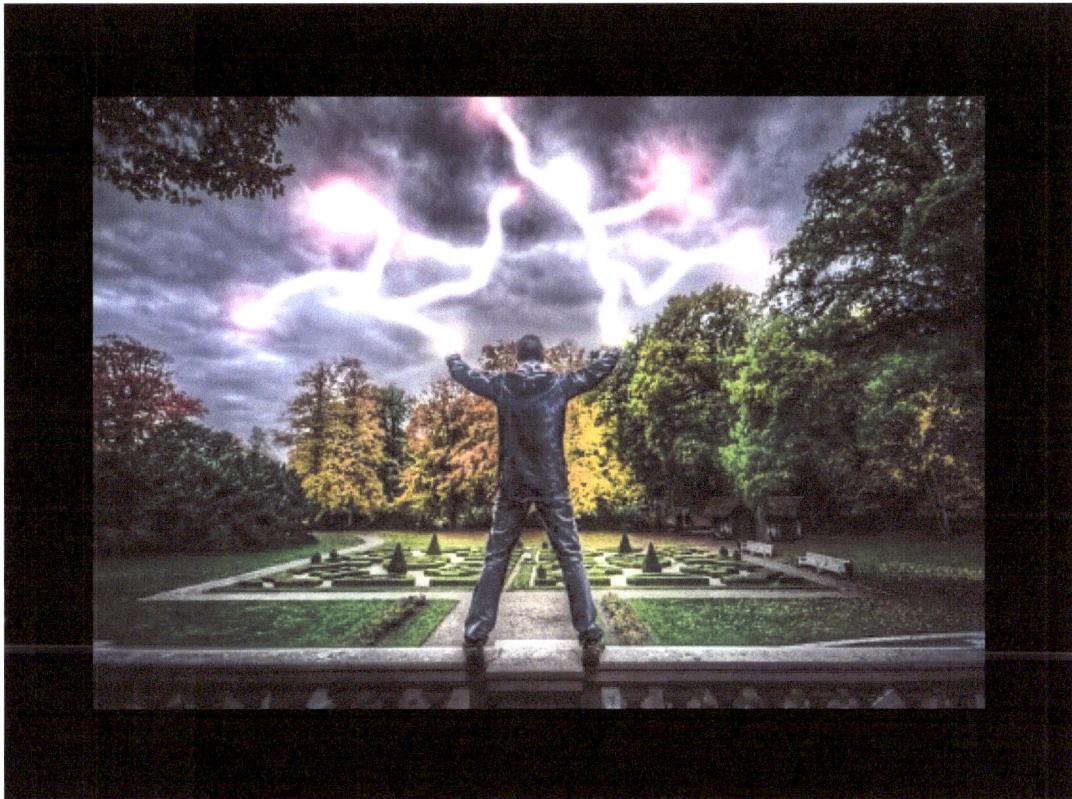

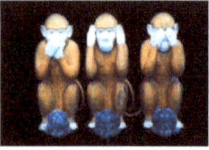

Step Three

Made a decision to turn our will and our lives over to the care of God as we understood Him.

Step three is simply a decision to live in the solution to addiction. Do you want to live in the problem or do you want to live in the solution? _____.

Think about all of the people, things, and circumstances that you have attempted to control in the past. What was the result? Do you think a Higher Power could handle things better than you? Y/N

Why?

_____.

Do you have fear about letting go and letting a Higher Power take over? _____

What fears do you have?

How do you plan to turn your will and your life over to the care of God as you understand Him?

_____

_____.

Who is God as you understand Him?

_____.

Who do you trust if anyone or anything?

_____.

What changes do you expect to make after letting go and letting God?

The Third Step Prayer is on Page 63 in **the Basic Text**, or "**Big Book**" of Alcoholics Anonymous. Many use the prayer when taking step three. The prayer is under the copyright of AA World Services, so I will not include it here.

Many in early recovery will say the prayer with their sponsors. The third step prayer seems to be very effective to serve the purpose of letting go and letting God take over. Most have wonderful results!

Everything that you do in the first three steps will prepare you for your fourth step. You must understand the disease of addiction, admit and accept that you have a problem in step one before you can find the solution in step two. In step two you find the solution to the disease of addiction, you learn to have a Higher Power of your understanding. You learn to let go and let God. In step three you make a decision to live in the solution to addiction or continue to live in the problem.

• Let's change things for a moment to give you a different perspective.

We are going to make up some symptoms of a disease that don't exist. Humor me, please.

Symptoms: Red Eyes, High Body Temperatures, Bumps on the skin, a limp in the left leg, and a cough. You have these symptoms, so you go to the Doctor, after running some tests, she says you have Meglaterglatitus. You know what the symptoms are, and you know what the disease is. The Doctor gives you a script for Plankton X 500. Now you have identified the solution to the disease.

You know the symptoms: Red Eyes, High Body Temperatures, Bumps on the skin, a limp in the left leg, and a cough. You know the disease or problem: Meglaterglatitus you know the solution: Plankton X 500

Are you getting better yet? Y/N Why?

_____.

You go to the pharmacy and get your script for Plankton X500 filled and take it home and put the bottle on your dresser. Are you getting better yet? Y/N Why?

_____.

You open the bottle of Plankton X500 and take it as the Doctor prescribes. Are you getting better yet? Y/N Why?

_____.

It's the same thing with addiction! You're not going to start to get better until you identify the problem and the solution, make a decision to live in the solution, and start to take the action to get well. That means you need to take step four if you want to start to change!

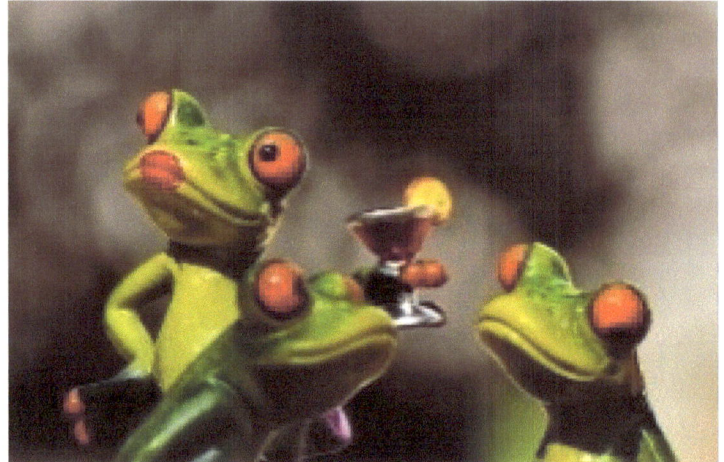

The best way to describe a decision is the old story of The Three Frogs!

There were three frogs perched up on a log in the swamp one day. One frog made a decision to jump off of the log. How many frogs were left on the log? _____.

The answer is three because the one frog only made a decision to jump off of the log, he didn't actually jump off. That is the essence of step three. This frog story has been used for decades to illustrate step three.

What does your will and your life mean to you?

_____.

To some, there will has been defined as their thinking and their lives as their actions. Pretty simple! Try reading step three using these two new words and meanings.
A. Are you convinced that if your life is run on self-will that it cannot be a success? Y/N
B. Are you convinced that you can't play God? Y/N
C. Are you convinced that God knows better than you? Y/N

"Half measures avail us nothing." In other words, we need to be committed if we want the miracle of recovery in our lives. The *"Basic Text"* says *"We are reborn"* meaning we change the way that we live and the way that we think. We experience an entire psychic change.

- The vehicle to change is the program and the twelve steps and the fellowship support that program of change.
- *"Next we launched out on a course of vigorous action"* from the *Basic Text* of AA.
- That means you immediately and aggressively start working on step four with your sponsor.
- The drugs and alcohol were but a symptom of the disease of addiction, step four will show the causes of the condition.

- Next, is step four the personal inventory: be honest and complete.
- Journaling/Prayer/Meditation becomes very important.

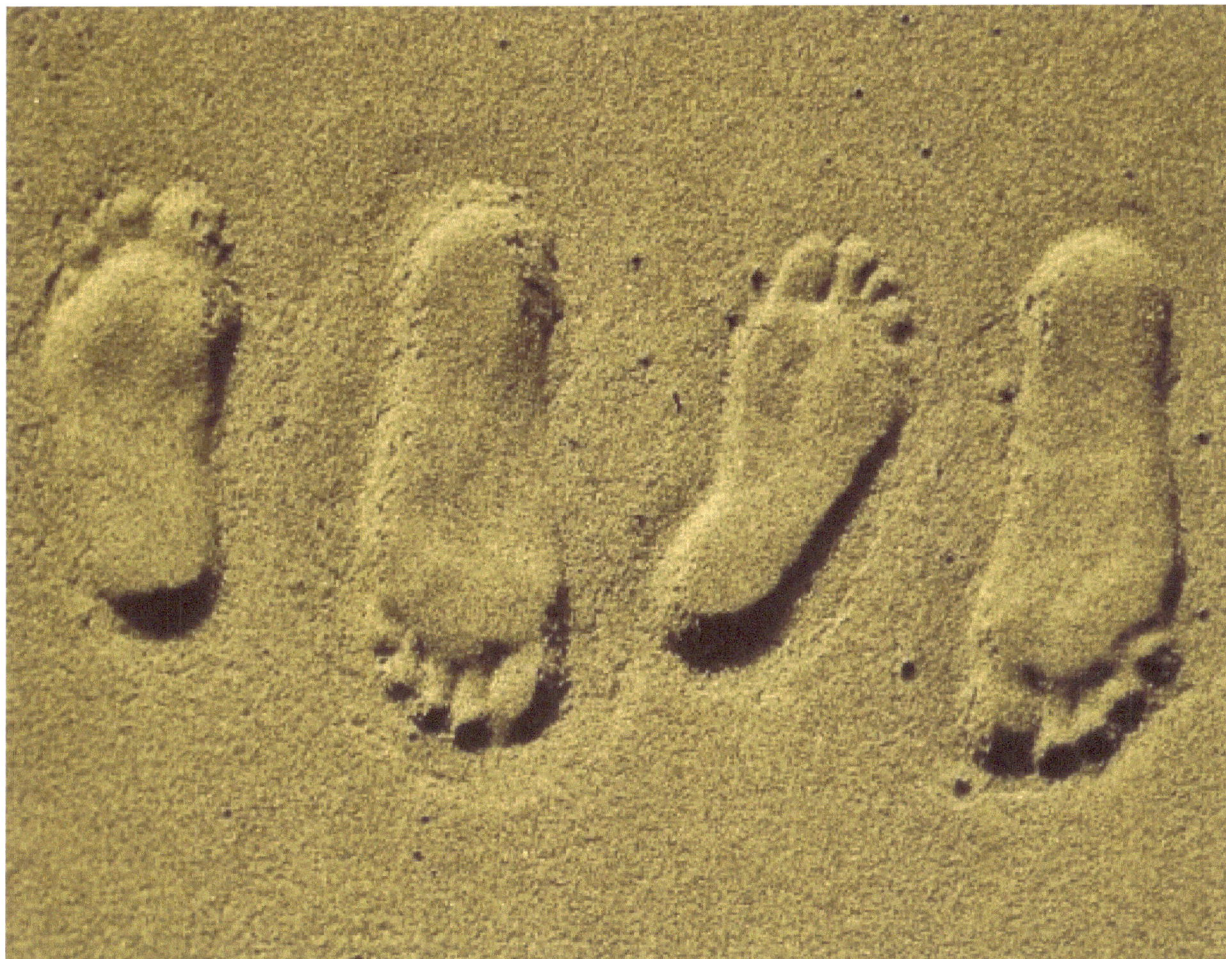

Step Four

Made a searching and fearless moral inventory of ourselves.

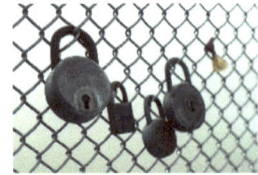

If you were a grocery store owner, you would have to take inventory of sellable and unsellable goods, or you would be out of business very quickly. Below is your imaginary grocery store: The Bell pepper and the carrots have gone bad.

What should you do?

_____.

The truth is if you don't get rid of the bad veggies, they will spoil the good ones. Keep that principle in mind as you do your personal inventory. The grocer has to be honest with himself. He can't cut corners. If he misses even one pepper or carrot that is bad, he puts all the others at risk.

Problem/ Solution/ Decision/ Program of Action/ Fellowship of Support

- Self-Acceptance comes before Self-Improvement!
- Our Problem = Lack of Power Centered in the Mind and triggered by the body.
- Our Solution = Take refuge in a Power Greater than any one of us, knowing we can be restored to sanity, and made whole.
- Our Decision = To live in that solution and Power one day at a time.
- Our Program of Action = to Turn our life and Will over to the Power and utilize the discipline of the twelve steps on a daily basis.
- Our Fellowship of Support = Our Fellowship supports the Program of Action with Sponsorship and Peers, Meetings, Sharing experience, Strength, and Hope.

Our 4TH Step is not designed to judge, but to identify problems so that we can change. A true and accurate picture of self and how we have been involved in real perspectives and proportions. Where have we been selfish, dishonest, self-seeking, inconsiderate, controlling and manipulative? Where had we been driven by fear in one form or another? We will find accurate descriptions of what has blocked us from our spirit. We will find a new perspective and a new way of life. We must avoid retaliation at all costs, and become willing to set all matters straight.

Think about anything that you are so ashamed of that it might block you from an honest step four. Who would it hurt if you told this? Can you work through this with someone you trust?

Is there anything else blocking you from being ready to do step four? Y/N
If Yes, What?

_____   _____.

We are going to take a look at the manifestations of self-will where the spirit is blocked by self-centeredness or harmful-self. We know that the basic instincts have become out of balance such as social, security, and sexual. Because of this in came fears, resentments, sexual harms, and other harms. We will look at these four categories and also list assets.

We write this down on paper using columns. We listed people, institutions, and principles.
I am resentful at the cause is because it affects my because I was.

Self	My Addiction	Everything	SDIFS

1. First list down the columns, list people, institutions, and principles. Your four lists will be:
A. Resentments
B. Fears
C. Sex Harms.
D. Other Harms

You will also do a fifth list that will be all of your assets: your good qualities.

2. The Cause: Why are you resentful, fearful, or did you cause harm?

3. What did it affect: Affects your self-esteem, financial, ambitions, relationships, sex relations, hurt or threatened, pride, security.

4. Where had you been fearful, selfish, self-seeking, or dishonest?

For the sex harms inventory list where had you been selfish, dishonest, inconsiderate, jealous, bitter, or suspicious?

5. Some like to do a fifth column: what could they have done differently?

• Remember the inventory is yours, not someone else's! Look for what you own, don't look to blame.
• Resentment they say is the number one offender! You must be rid of anger.
• Fear is also a problem. Faith takes care of fear. We outgrow fear over time.
• Harms the other problem will stop as you start to live a spirit-centered life.

The Original Way of doing Step Four is as Follows:

List real resentments:
Column 1: In dealing with resentments we set them on paper. We listed people, institutions or principles with whom we were angry.

Column 2: We asked ourselves why we were angry.

Column 3: On our grudge list we set opposite each name our injuries. Was it our self-esteem, our security, our ambitions, our personal, or sex relations that had been interfered with?

Column 4: Referring to our list again. Putting out of our minds the wrongs others had done, we resolutely looked for our own mistakes. Where had we been selfish, dishonest, self-seeking and frightened?

Column 5: This Column is optional. List specific other defects to show your participation in the resentments.

Reading from left to right we now see the resentment (**Column 1**), the cause (**Column 2),** the part of self that had been affected.

(**Column 3**) and the exact nature of the defect within us that allowed the resentment to surface and block us off from God's will.

(Columns 4 and 5):
Complete each column top to bottom before proceeding to the next column. Thus, for instance, fill in all the names of those you are resentful at theoretical resentments. Is the resentment a problem for you, does it cause you pain?

Column 3 Col. 4 Column 5:
Affects My Specific
Mistakes (optional)
Own Defects

> You can make your own chart or use one that is already made. Remember to list down the first column then across. There are a total of five Inventories:

1. Resentments
2. Fears
3. Sex Harms
4. Other Harms
5. Assets or positive qualities

Sex Harms
Complete each column top to bottom before going on to the next column.

- **Column 1:** We reviewed our sex conduct over the years past. Whom had we hurt?
- **Column 2:** Where had we been selfish, dishonest, or inconsiderate?
- **Column 3:** Did we unjustifiably arouse jealousy, suspicion, or bitterness?
- **Column 4:** Where were we at fault?
- **Column 5**: What should we have done instead?

Assets:

List all of the good qualities about yourself.

Sex Inventory Chart (example)

One   Two   Three   Four   Five

Who Hurt	S.D.I.	J.S.B.	Fault	Instead
Me	SDI	JSB	My Own	Minded Own

Fears:

Complete column 1 from top to bottom before proceeding to the next column.

• **Column 1:** We reviewed our fears thoroughly. We put them on paper, even though we had no resentment in connection with them.
• **Column 2**: We asked ourselves why we had them. Be realistic. Discuss significant fears, not theoretical or imaginary fears.

I'm Fearful of:	Why Do I Have the Fear?

Harms Other:

Who Hurt	S.D.I.	J.S.B.	Fault	Instead

Assests	Liabilities
Humility	Self-justification
Modesty	Procrastination
Self-valuation	Resentment
Honesty	Self-pity
Patience	Hate
Love	Impatience
Forgiveness	Self-importance

Can you think of any others?

Assests	8.	Liabilities	8.
1.	9.	1.	9.
2.	10.	2.	10.
3.	11.	3.	11.
4.	12.	4.	12.
5.	13.	5.	13.
6.	14.	6.	14.
7.	15.	7.	15.

What part of us was disturbed by others? This often relates to feelings associated with our attitudes, behaviors, and personalities in reaction to any threats to our basic instincts. (Security/Self Esteem/Sex/Relationship)

Where are we responsible? Where have we been selfish, self-seeking, dishonest, inconsiderate, or driven by fear? Where have we manipulated and not thought of others? In step four we get accurate descriptions on what has blocked us from the spirit.

Changing our lives. In focused prayer and meditation, we realize that others are also sick and suffering. We pray for help for others and ourselves for healing body, mind, and spirit. We join the human race once again, no longer an island that the World revolves around.

Remember that step four is a fact-finding and fact-facing process. It is a personal inventory to find damaged and undamaged goods. (Assets and liabilities) Let the change and healing begin!

Don't be a fool about values!

Step Five

Admitted to God, to ourselves, and to another human being the exact nature of our wrongs.

> You are going to want to be very careful who you choose to share your 4TH step with! Remember some are sicker than others! You don't have to do your 5TH step with your program sponsor. You can do your 5TH step with a trusted friend, clergy member, family member, counselor, etc. Just make sure that you trust them.

After step four is completed: what have you learned about your limitations and capabilities?_____
_____.

Make a list of the people that you think that you can share your 4TH and 5TH step with below:

Person's Names	Safe, risky, or no

Pick the person that you will do step five with?_____.

Set a date and time to do your 5TH step with your chosen trusted person.___/___/_____ ____: _____
Fifth Step to be completed.

Pick a quiet location where you will not be disturbed during the process of your step work.
Keep the commitment and get the step done.

Describe what it was like sharing your Fifth Step with your "HP" and another person:
_____
_____.

Describe any activities or celebrations that you did in honor of completing your Fifth Step:

Describe how you felt the moment you completed your Fifth Step in the boxes below:

CONGRATULATIONS!

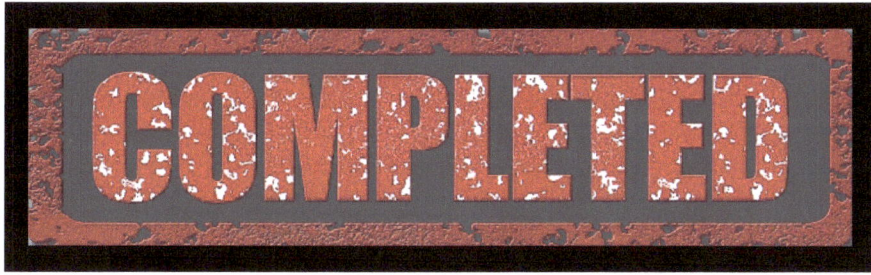

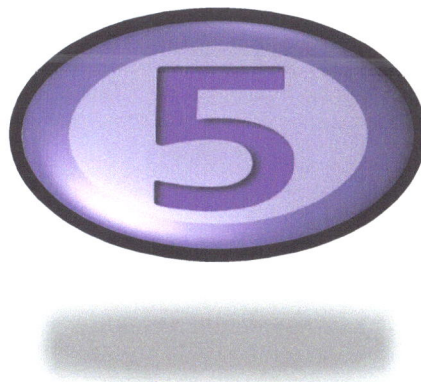

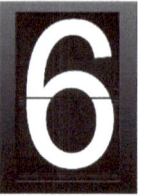

Step Six

I become entirely ready to have God remove all of these defects of character.

Describe some activities that you really enjoy doing:

List some selfish acts that you have done in the box below:

List some good deeds that you have done in the box below:

List Your Major Character Defects in the Box below:

List Your Assets in the Box below:

What do you plan to do when these major character defects arise? List each major character defect individually along with a preventative behavior and how you are willing to allow God to help you:

(Use the back of the sheet if the box is not large enough.)

Are you ready to have God take control of these behaviors and attitudes? Y/N

List some good deeds that you would like to do:

Step Seven

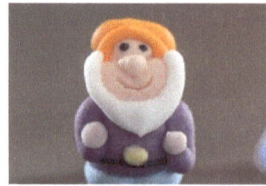

I humbly ask God to remove my shortcomings.

What defects will be the most difficult for you to surrender:

What are your Triggers for regression back into your old character defects?

Examples			
Stress			
Fear			
Anger			
Not enough sleep			

What makes you lose hope and how can you avoid this?

_____.

Is there a situation, person, or place that gives you hope? Y/N

How can you maximize this influence; fill in the boxes below:

What have you lost in your life because of addiction that you would like to get back in recovery?

When your character defects are removed, what do you think your new life will be like?

Wonderful	Beautiful	Unchanged	A Miracle

Please list the things that you are grateful for as of today:

What do you want your legacy to be? Fill in the boxes below:

Write your name here and describe yourself in the boxes below:
Name: _____.

Draw a picture that describes how you feel:

Step Eight

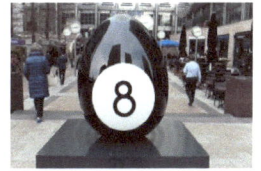

I make a list of persons that I have harmed and become willing to make amends to them all.

Make a list of all the people including yourself that were harmed because of your addiction, the effects on your relationships and them as individuals.

People Harmed:	Effects on Relationship:	Effects on Individuals:

Use back of page if more room needed.

Next, make a list of possible Amends for each person harmed:

Person Harmed:	Possible Amends:

Use back of page if more room needed.

What possible consequence could happen as a result of making the Amends:

Person Harmed:	Possible Amends:	Possible Consequence:

Do you have any resentments toward anyone on your amends list? Y/N
If you do, how can you handle it?

_____.

Do you have any fear in making amends to anyone on your amends list? Y/N
If yes, what can you do:

_____ .

Describe any other blocks that you may have to making amends when the proper time comes:

_____ .

Do you feel that you are ready to make amends when the opportunity presents itself? Y/N
Explain your answer:

_____ .

On a scale of one to ten, ten being the most confident, how confident do you feel about making amends?_____.

Step Nine

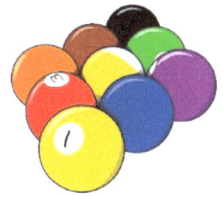

I make direct amends to such people whenever possible, except when to do so would injure them or others.

It's important not to rush amends and not to do them when you're not ready! Amends need to be done on God's timing when you have worked with your sponsor and are prepared. There's nothing worse than a premature amends, and then a relapse and you lose all credibility. You have to be prepared before you execute!

When you make an amends, never tell the other person what you think they did wrong. Just own what you did wrong.

Role-playing situations with your sponsor trusted friends, and family can help you to prepare for the real amends.

It would be wise to keep a log of your amends, what works for you, what doesn't work, what you should do differently, etc.

Remember that some people may not forgive you! That's Okay! This is about you keeping your side of the street clean. Others can do what they want. Some people will surprise you. The ones that you thought would never forgive you may be the first ones to forgive you. You never know how people are going to react? The important thing is that you do the next right thing in your recovery. Don't let fear keep you from doing what is right.

Some people may say some hard things that you don't want to hear about your past. You will have to be prepared to take their worst without retaliation.

Remember what this step says: make direct amends to such people whenever possible, except when to do so would injure them or others. Read the second half of this carefully and use good common sense. Don't place anyone in harm's way!

If you have committed a crime and making amends will expose you to arrest, you have the right to consult an attorney. If it's of a serious nature that would be wise. (We are not lawyers and are not comfortable to give advice in this area)

Do you think that you are prepared to make direct amends to those you have harmed during your addiction? Y/N

Comments: _____.

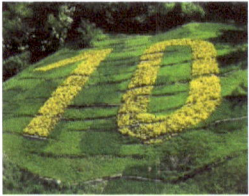

Step Ten

I continue to take personal inventory, and when I am wrong I promptly admit it.

There are Three Types of Inventories:
1. Step Four: Major Personal Inventory
2. Daily Inventory: when we retire at night we constructively review our day.
3. Spot Inventory: when we're wrong, we promptly admit it.

How do you plan to reflect on your day?

_____.

What Triggers do you need to watch out for?

What New Behaviors will make your program more effective:

How will you implement these New Behaviors?

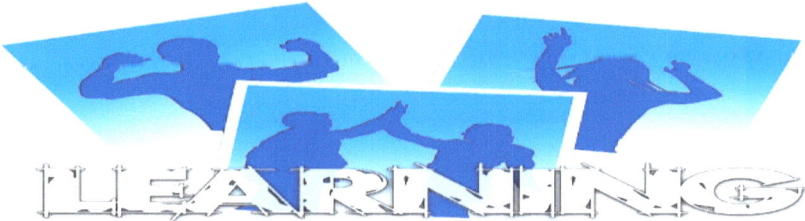

Step Eleven

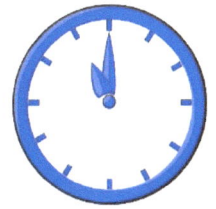

Through prayer and meditation, I seek to improve my conscious contact with God as I understand God, praying only for knowledge of God's will for my life and the power to carry that out.

How would you describe prayer?

How would you describe meditation?

How would you define a belief?

Where did you learn about healthy values, wisdom, and knowledge?

What do you think God's will is for you in this life?

Did you ever turn your life and will over to anyone or anything else besides God in your lifetime? Y/N
If yes, what or who:

What would you want your obituary to say? Write in the box:

Do you ever meditate? Y/N
If yes, how:

How can you improve your conscious contact with God as you understand Him?

What do you think happens to you after you pass?

In the Box Draw, a Picture of Your Higher Power as He or She would look today in your mind.

How can you improve your relationship with the Divine?
Write your answers in the boxes below:

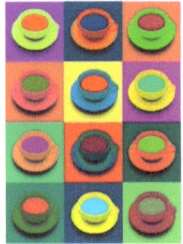

Step Twelve

Having had a spiritual awakening as the result of these steps, I try to carry this message to others and to practice these principles in all of my life.

Please describe what a Spiritual Awakening means to you:

_____
_____.

How important do you think it is to have "Sober Time" to sponsor others in early recovery?

1 least	2	3	4	5	6	7	8	9	10 tops

Do you think Twelve-Step Programs Work? Y/N
Why?

How do you plan to carry the message?

Do you believe that Anonymous means that you can't tell people that you're in recovery? Y/N
Why?

_____.

How do you plan to practice these principles in all your affairs?

They say that you have to give it away if you want to keep it! Please list ways that you will do service work and give back:

Chair Meetings			

Random Acts of Kindness that are only between you and your "HP" are a great way to give back and be spiritual. Please list some random acts of kindness that you can do, I'll list a few to get you started:

Pay someone's toll			
Pay someone's Meter			
Wash Someone's car			
Pay someone's check			
Mow elderly lawn			
Flowers to neighbor			
Gift nursing home			
Groceries needy			

There are so many wonderful things that you can do each day, and it doesn't have to involve money. It could be as simple as a well-placed smile, and you could make someone else's day.

It's all about thoughts, attitudes, choices, decisions, and actions! Who do you want to be? You have a choice today.

You are no longer bound by the burden of the chains of self-centeredness, you are free! The truth sets us, free friends. You have worked through the twelve steps and discovered the truth about yourself. You have learned about your disease, the solution to your disease, made a decision to live in that solution, taken the action steps to change, the growth and maintenance steps to continue to change, and been supported by a wonderful fellowship in the process.

Congratulations, as the "*Big Book*" says, "*you are reborn*" you have had an entire psychic change in the way that you live and the way that you think. You are a new creation!

Wisdom

Read the first 164 pages of *"**The Big Book**"* as soon as possible in recovery that gives you the entire program.

Get a sponsor as soon as possible, not a family member or friend; someone that will call you on your defects and help you work the steps.

"You are not alone."

You are not terminally unique!
Whatever your problems are, someone else has made it through with the same problems at some point.
A sponsor is a guide to the steps, not a banker, counselor, etc.
Meeting makers make it is a half-truth, they make it if they work it!
The stories in the back of *"**The Big Book**"* are to identify not compare.
Get an address book and get names and numbers at meetings, some day you will need every name and number in the book!
Don't go to major events like weddings and funerals alone; take someone else in recovery with you.
Alcoholics don't go to bars to listen to the piano player!
If you hang around the barn long enough, you will get hay on you!

"Don't hang around slippery people, places, and things!"

Those corny sayings are life-saving like *"One day at a time!"*
"Insanity is doing the same thing over and over again and expecting different results."

"Denial is not a river in Egypt!"

The Twelve Steps would benefit anyone!

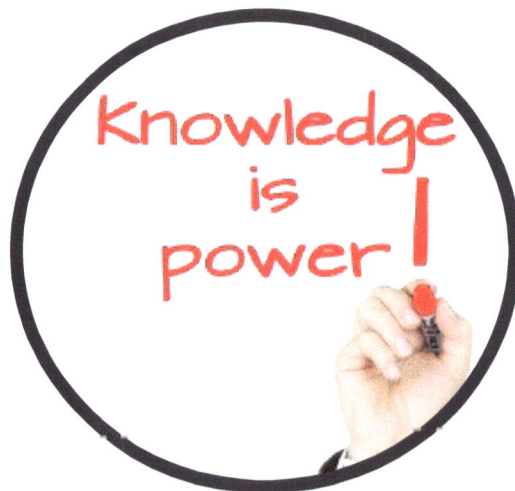

Action Planning:

Action plans need to be specific.
Identify Goals and Objectives.
How do you get from point A. to point B.?
Who is going to assist you?
Why do you need to do this action?
Where are you going to do this action?
What is the plan?
Who will follow-up?
On what timetable, be specific?

Example:

Goals and Objectives:	To Improve Communication with coworkers
How:	Clarify Expectations, Meetings
Why:	To Improve Teamwork and Consistency
Who:	John Clarify Expectations, Everyone at Meetings
Where:	XYZ Corp. Meeting Room
When:	Friday, August 22, 2014, 4PM.
Follow Up:	John and Coach
Details of the plan:	Keep Notes, Memos, Daily Info Log, Meeting Minutes, Training for Employees, Employee Manual.

Can be short or long-term: 30 Days, 6 Months, 1 Year, etc.

Below is a blank Action Plan for you to copy and use as a template (On the next page)

Remember, successful people create great Action Plans and follow through with them.

Action Plans

Goals and Objectives: **Specific Dates:**

Action: **Specific Dates:**

Follow-Up Plan: **Specific Dates:**

➢ What, how, when, who, why, what? Be specific!
➢ Substance Abuser sets goals and objectives. Sponsor or Coach and Substance Abuser work on an action plan.
➢ The plan may have to be adjusted is something is not working, be flexible.

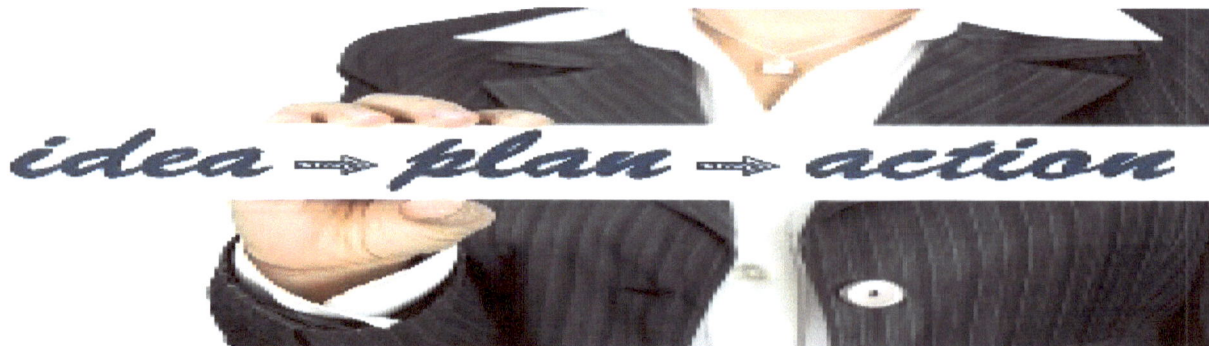

Anger Log

Date	Angry at?	Why I am angry and what I did about it? (positive or negative behavior.)	P/N

Activities

Activities to work on in early Recovery:

Write out your life story and at the same time do a timeline of the major events that happened in your life both positive and negative.

Journaling every day, you are basically keeping a diary as you go through early recovery. It's important that you make entries in the morning and when you retire at night. Look to see where you can improve in your thinking and the way that you live.

Make a gratitude list, at least, twenty things every day.

Write an Anger Log, you have a blank form in this manual. Learn to identify signs and symptoms of anger, where your anger comes from: where is your hurt and fear coming from? Learn to deal with angry feelings in a constructive way like writing or lifting weights, before the behavior turns destructive.

Learn to use the 500 lb. telephone and call your sponsor, recovery coach, and other recovering people. When you share your burden, it becomes much lighter. Buy a small address book and get at least three new names and phone numbers at every meeting that you go to, someday you will need them, trust me!

Make an Action Plan with your recovery coach or sponsor. The information, instructions, and templates are in the manual.

Exercise and eat right. Check with your doctor to make sure that you're healthy enough for the form of exercise that you want to do. Get on a well-balanced diet, when is the last time you ate three square meals a day?

Avoid "Slippery people, places, and things!" "Stick with the winners!" Find fun clean and sober activities that you enjoy: writing, weight lifting, reading, walking, running, sports, etc.
"Move a muscle, change a thought!" If you are struggling, stay busy. If you sit around and get into your head, you're in trouble, please, stay busy! Volunteer at non-profits, soup kitchens, nursing homes, animal shelters, homeless shelters, give back where you can.

Do service work, take all the service commitments that you can find, at meetings and outside of meetings. Help the old lady next door who can't rake her own leaves, fix her fence, take a coffee commitment, speak at meetings.

Learn to tell on yourself when you're in a bad space, it might just save your life, or someone else's.

Remember that meeting makers make it, if they work it. You have to do the footwork. Get a sponsor right away, read the first 164 pages in the Basic Text of AA, do step work, etc.

Prayer and Meditation are important and go a long way.

Remember that you're not alone!

Resources

Dual Recovery Anonymous: http://draonline.org/
Heroin Anonymous:
http://www.heroin-anonymous.org/haws/index.html.
Marijuana Anonymous: http://www.marijuana-anonymous.org/.
Methadone Anonymous Support:
http://www.methadonesupport.org/.
Narcotics Anonymous: http://www.na.org/.
Nar-anon:
http://www.nar-anon.org/Nar-Anon/Nar-Anon_Home.html
Nicotine Anonymous: http://www.nicotine-anonymous.org/.
Pills Anonymous: http://www.pillsanonymous.org/.
Sober 24: http://www.sober24.com/
Adult Children of Alcoholics (ACOA):
http://www.adultchildren.org/
Al-Anon; Al-Ateen: http://www.al-anon.alateen.org/
Alcoholics Anonymous: http://www.aa.org/.
Cocaine Anonymous: http://www.ca.org/.
Crystal Meth Anonymous: http://www.crystalmeth.org/.
Double Trouble in Recovery:
http://www.doubletroubleinrecovery.org/
The National Council on Problem Gambling
730 11th St, NW, Ste 601
Washington, DC 20001
Phone 202.547.9204
Fax 202.547.9206
1-800-522-4700 Helpline
ncpg@ncpgambling.org

It Takes a Village!

There is a saying in the rooms of twelve-step recovery programs, "The definition of insanity is doing the same thing over and over and expecting different results!" Sometimes I wonder if they're talking about the pathology of addiction of describing the current paradigm of treatment. Short-term treatment is not effective. This is not an attempt to condemn or pass blame; it is an attempt to find better solutions to an insidious disease. Our young are dying in record numbers there must be a more effective solution to the problem.

In the fall of 1968, a seven-year-old boy accompanied his mother to a meeting of Alcoholics Anonymous, the room was filled with smoke, every table had an ashtray filled with extinguished cigarettes, and most of the people were middle-aged. The people were very friendly, and there were many smiles and lots of chatter. The chairperson banged down the gavel, and the meeting started. The preamble of AA was read by one of the men and then the twelve steps of AA. Then the speaker began to tell his story. The mother gave her son a dollar to put in a wicker basket that was passed to help satisfy the AA tradition that the meeting is self-supporting. There were coffee and cookies on a table in the back of the room for all to enjoy. The speaker talked for about forty-five minutes and then others at the meeting shared until the hour was nearly over. The meeting closed with the group holding hands in a large circle and chanting "The Lord's Prayer."

The mother enjoyed over forty years of continuous sobriety until she passed on a few years ago. The boy had yet to start his "addiction career" at that time of his life. Later in his life, he returned to the rooms of AA, not to accompany another, but for his own sake. Sobriety was short-lived. There were to be three trips to residential treatment to an AA rest farm started by one of the co-founders of AA, Bill W. There were no doctors or nurses, just a professional staff of other recovering alcoholics who cared.
The first two times to the farm, the man didn't listen, was self-centered, and didn't take the suggestions of the staff or the program of AA. The third visit to the farm was different; the man was as willing as the dying could be. He got honest, was open-minded, and took every suggestion and put them into action.

The man is still enjoying continuous sobriety of approximately eighteen years to date. The man's brother and his brother's wife also found recovery in the rooms of AA and a twelve-step rest farm. The couple has been clean and sober for approximately sixteen years to date. The man's uncle also found hope in AA and has enjoyed thirty years of continuous sobriety to date. Five people, in one family, who all found the miracle of long-term recovery. Why do so many others fail?

In today's recovery world, experience and science have shown us that the addicted person's family must also be addressed, not just the addicted person. Addiction has proven itself to be a family disease. Not necessarily that more than one person in the family is addicted, but the whole family is affected by the disease. The family needs to understand addiction and recovery so that they can support recovery without enabling addiction. They need to be educated as to the true pathology of addiction. The problem defines the solution. There are no short cuts; there is no easier way out. I heard someone say the other day, "It takes a village" to help the addict to recover.

Think about the facts. How do most people start off recovery? If they're willing to get help, they go to detox, if not they have an intervention, or take more lumps. Then they go to a short-term stay in a residential program. (Less than 90 days.) A professional drives the process. Then there is total disengagement.

The family may not even communicate with anyone else but their addicted family member. Their loved one returns home, and the family thinks that their loved one is cured. Does this sound familiar and about right? This process doesn't work! Treatment works, the process does not.

Let's look at some of the problems. Not every person that needs help gets help. More than 50% of the people who go for treatment don't stay to complete the program, and their families enable them. Only a small minority get continuing care. Most people don't get a long enough stay for initial treatment. Most people relapse within a year of treatment, those that consume alcohol and other drugs relapse within 90 days. Those that have a high rate of recovery and low rate of relapse get there at between four and five years of remission. The professionals have all disengaged with the addicted person when they need more help.

How did the family mentioned earlier have five successful long-term recoveries? What worked for them? The first fact is that the family was educated in addiction and recovery because the mother took the family to open AA meetings. The whole family heard about supporting recovery and not enabling. They also heard speakers talk about the reality of addiction. They knew that less than ninety days in a residential program would not give them a solid foundation to build a sober life upon. They had continued coaching from family and friends in recovery. They learned from each other's mistakes. The family acted as case managers for each other. The family opened a non-medical residential addiction recovery program modeled after the program that the first son attended. The family had aftercare. I guess it did take a small village for a successful recovery!

Based on my training and observation, it is my opinion that the recovery world is about to undergo a major paradigm shift in addiction recovery treatment. There has to be more focus on post-treatment. There needs to be continuing education for the whole family of those suffering from addiction, professionals, peers, and those addicted. Everyone needs to have a coach! Recovery coaches for those addicted, family recovery coaches for the families. The whole process needs to be results and client driven. There needs to be case managers externally from treatment programs that monitor from assessment to disengagement that should not conclude prior to five years. Early re-intervention when needed.

Just like everyone links up to social media, those addicted will need to link up with recovery communities. We also need to continue to develop community recovery resources, learning as we go. Give more credibility to those with years of addiction recovery, they know what works and what doesn't. Give reasonable choices to those addicted in different modalities.

Addiction treatment and recovery isn't as simple as just not using illicit drugs and alcohol. Recovery is about changing the way that the person thinks and lives. Recovery is a lifetime commitment. It's about saying yes to life and doing the next right thing. Recovery is a gift to the hopeless and dying. We all need to work together for a better future. Recovery is as much about the spirit as it is about the mind and body. Science alone will never find the answer, nor will religion, or government policy makers. It will take the whole village! One last thing, if you were wondering, yes I am that boy!

Sources: (Jin 98) (Wilbourne & Miller 02) (Hubbard, Flynn, Haddock, Fletcher 01) (Godly & Dennis 01) (SAMHSA 03)
Rev. Dr. K.T. Coughlin Ph.D.
www.theaddiction.expert

The Twelve Steps

Twelve-Step Recovery Slogans: *"Keep it Green, Live and Let Live, Think, Think, Think, Easy Does it, keep It Simple, One Day at a Time, There but for the Grace of God Go I, Let Go and Let God. Meeting Makers Make it, if They Work it, You are Not Alone, First Things First, This too Shall Pass, Expect Miracles, Stick with the Winners."* *These slogans are life savers!*

There Are Twelve Promises That Come With The Twelve Steps

The Twelve Promises

1. If we are painstaking about this phase of our development, we will be amazed before we are half way through.
2. We are going to know a new freedom and a new happiness.
3. We will not regret the past nor wish to shut the door on it.
4. We will comprehend the word serenity and we will know peace.
5. No matter how far down the scale we have gone, we will see how our experience can benefit others.
6. That feeling of uselessness and self-pity will disappear.
7. We will lose interest in selfish things and gain interest in our fellows.
8. Self-seeking will slip away.
9. Our whole attitude and outlook upon life will change.
10. Fear of people and of economic insecurity will leave us.
11. We will intuitively know how to handle situations which used to baffle us.
12. We will suddenly realize that God is doing for us what we could not do for ourselves.

Are these extravagant promises? We think not. (AA and other Twelve-Step fellowships) These Twelve Promises will come True if we work for them; they did for me!

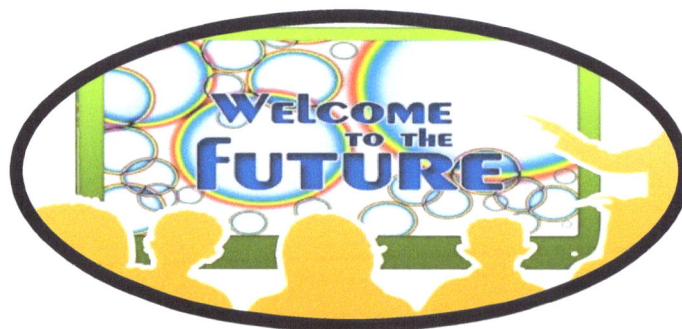

Albert

"Hi, my name is Albert," the awkward little man said, as he waddled down the church sidewalk. His face was wrinkled, and his hair was gray. He wore an old suit from decades past. There were food and coffee stains all down the front of his shirt, tie, and blazer. The clothes didn't fit quite right.

You could tell that Albert had mental health issues at first glance. His outstretched hand was shaking as he waited to clasp on to mine. His words were hurried and difficult to understand. Albert was as friendly as a puppy that just found a new home. He was a very gentle, yet enthusiastic soul.

It turned out that Albert was assigned to service work at the Friday night twelve-step meeting. His job was to greet people as they came for the meeting at 8:00 PM. Albert lived in a home, not far from the church. In the meeting, when it was time for people to share, Albert raised his hand up high and said, "My name is Albert, and I'm an alcoholic!" He repeated that same mantra, week after week for years. He would always faithfully be there on the sidewalk to greet newcomers.

At first, I thought Albert was very strange. After a couple of weeks, I looked forward to Albert's greetings. He would light up, like a Christmas tree whenever he greeted anyone. He really would make people feel welcome. He was as important as any other part of the meeting each week. He was full of love, care, and compassion. It was not unusual for Albert to have fresh cookie crumbs and coffee on his shirt and tie.

For years, Albert only said the same mantra, "My name is Albert, and I'm an alcoholic!" He said nothing more, and nothing less. I don't know his actual age, but he must have been in his late seventies or older. After many years, Albert decided that he would take on the Friday night meeting speaking commitment. Everyone was amazed, because, for years, all we ever heard him say was, "My name is Albert, and I'm an alcoholic!" The very next Friday night meeting, Albert was the keynote speaker. He went on for almost an hour. He kept everyone entertained, as he talked about his battle with alcoholism and his many years of recovery. Albert's personal story was delivered in an eloquent manner. Many of the people at the meeting were touched by the speech; some were in tears. You could tell that Albert was very pleased as he shook hands with everyone after the meeting.

That night Albert returned to the home. He died of a massive heart attack in his sleep. The meeting was never quite the same. Although every time I got out of my car at the church, I could still see the vision of old Albert rumbling down the sidewalk to greet me. There are no coincidences, they say. Albert finally shared his story, during his last night on Earth. Heaven is going to be interesting! I'm going to guess that when newcomers arrive, they will hear, "Hi, my name is Albert!"

Notes:

Rev. Dr. Kev.'s Publication Credits

KTC Phase IIC Coaching, LLC,2016 Book: *Addictions: What Parents Need to Know to Survive the Drug Epidemic*

KTC Phase IIC Coaching, LLC, 2015 Book: *In the Sunlight of the Spirit* Workbook & Guide

KTC Phase IIC Coaching, LLC, 2015 Book: *If You Want What We Have*; 12-Step Workbook & Guide

The Aurorean, Encircle Publications 1998 Poetry and Essays

Joel's House Publications 1998-2005 Poetry and Essays

Our Journey 1998-2005 Poetry

The Poetry Explosion, The Pen 1999-2003 Poetry

Apostrophe 1998 Poetry

Nuthouse Twin Rivers Press 1998 Poetry

The National Library of Poetry 1998

Lines N' Rhymes 1998 Poetry

The Poetry Church Feather Books

England. Anthology John Hunt Publications 1999 Poetry

A Tapestry in Time. 1999 Poetry Book 18 Poems

Connecticut Department of Mental Health and Addiction Services

The Webster Times 1999 Poetry

The Angel News 1999 Poetry

The Skater won The Editor's Choice Award September 1999 (Our Journey)

The Blind Man's Rainbow 1999 Poetry

Arnazella 2001 Poetry

Feather Books, The Poetry Church 1998-2002

The American Dissident 2002 Poetry

The Good Shepherd Poetry 2002

Ya ' Sou Magazine Essays and Poetry

Colt. Winner Editor's Choice Award Contest Literally Horses 2002

Goodbye My Friend Read on the Radio Rhyme and Reason UBC Europe & the UK

September 2001 Read on the Radio in Europe and the UK as a Tribute to those lost on September 11th bombings. My poem was read over the radio for many days.

Tumbleweed Read on BBC Radio in England 2001

Published by Feather Books

Notified by John Waddington Feather that Tumbleweed had been read on BBC Radio in England on Several Occasions.

Stanwich Congregational Flyer Poetry

University of Scranton Panuska College of Professionals Essay 2002

Scranton University 2002 Poetry

Tumbleweeds; Feather Books Poetry Series; A Book of Poetry Written by Rev. Kevin T. Coughlin Feather Books England May 2002 Rev. John Waddington Feather Founder (In Memory of DeWitt)

The River Reporter Newspaper 2002 Poetry

Unity Community News 2002 Poetry

The Poetry Corner Angelfire.com Poetry

The Poet's Market 2002 Poetry

The Poetry Church England 2003 Poetry

Cover of Wayne Independent News 2003 Poetry

Nomad's Choir 2003 Poetry

Written a series of 9 course manuals for a coaching recovery curriculum. 2014-2015

www.addictedminds.org 2015 Articles Matthew Steiner Founder

www.soberservices.com 2015 Articles

http://fromaddict2advocate.blogspot 2015 Articles Marilyn Davis Founder

Contentwriter.com Articles 2015-2016

LinkedIn 2014-2016 Articles
Two Drops of Ink S.W. Biddulph 2015 Poetry
The Addict's Mom 2015 Articles Blog
Ghostwriter Articles/ Content 2014-2015
CBS News Channel 10
NBC KHQ Q6 News
NBC Eyewitness News 8 KLKN TV
Fox 14 News at 9
Wayne Independent Newspaper Honesdale, PA
News Eagle, Hawley, PA
Reading Eagle, Reading, PA Berks & Beyond
Blog Talk Radio The Broken Brain
www.eatingdisorderhope.com

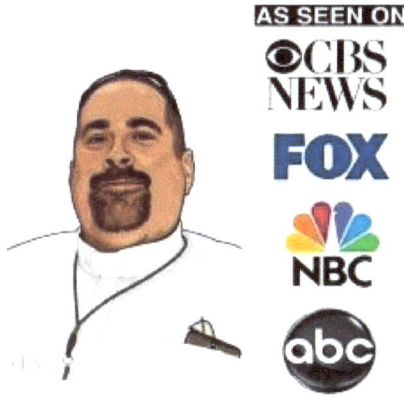

About The Author

Rev. Dr., Kevin T. Coughlin Ph.D., is a Master Coach, trainer, writer, poet, speaker, a Diplomate Christian counselor and therapist, he is Board Certified in Family, Developmental, Alcoholism, Substance Abuse, and Grief Counseling, the Reverend is a NCIP interventionist, a Domestic Violence Advocate, Associate Professor for DCU, a Provincial Superintendent (to be consecrated a Bishop in the Spring of 2016) and so much more; he is an expert in the field of Addiction and Recovery. He is the President and CEO of Phase IIC Coaching, LLC., and The Program Director for The Addictions Academy. The Reverend has over forty-seven years of experience with the AA program. He has been working in the addiction recovery field for almost two decades, has helped thousands of individuals and their families overcome all types of addictions, substance abuse, alcoholism, process addiction, shame and guilt, relationship and communication problems, anger management, inner healing, self-image, interventions and much more. He is a published author and has published thousands of poems and articles published throughout the United States and other Nations, he has been interviewed on numerous radio talk shows and published in magazines, newspapers, books, and online publications.

Thank you for reading my work! If you enjoyed my twelve-step workbook, would you consider reviewing it on Amazon.com? I would appreciate your help in getting the word out on how helpful this manual is in both understanding and working the twelve-step program. Thank you so much!
Best of life!

Rev. Dr. Kev.

Rev. Dr. Kev's Social Media Accounts

Facebook
1. Kevin Coughlin: https://www.facebook.com/profile.php?id=100008449955607
2. My Group, Resources for those suffering from addiction and their families: https://www.facebook.com/groups/resourcesforthosesufferingfromaddiction/
3. RevKev The Addiction Expert: https://www.facebook.com/RevKev/?fref=ts

Linkedin
1. Rev. Dr. Kevin T. Coughlin PhD https://www.linkedin.com/in/revkevnetwork

Google+
1. Kevin Coughlin https://plus.google.com/112400908736308001821/posts

My Group: The Recovery Community Family and Friends: https://plus.google.com/communities/113521225141112811207

Pinterest
1. Kevin Coughlin: https://www.pinterest.com/ktc1961/
2. My Group Board: Recovery We Can https://www.pinterest.com/ktc1961/recovery-we-can/

Tumblr
1. https://www.tumblr.com/blog/revkevsrecoveryworld

Instagram
theaddiction.expert

My Websites:
1. www.revkevsrecoveryworld.com
2. theaddiction.expert
3. theaddiction.guru

Rev. Dr. Kev's Goodreads Link: https://www.goodreads.com/author/show/14874631.Kevin_Coughlin
About.me Link: https://about.me/ktc1961/
http://ilikeebooks.com/if-you-want-what-we-have/
http://awesomegang.com
www.amazon.com/Rev.-Kevin-T-Coughlin/e/B01AF6AAAI/ref=ntt_dp_epwbk_0
http://mybookplace.net/in-the-sunlight-of-the-spirit-a-spirituality-training-manual-and-workbook-by-kevin-coughlin/

Thank you for reading my work! If you enjoyed my twelve-step workbook, would you consider reviewing it on Amazon.com? I would appreciate your help in getting the word out on how helpful this manual is in both understanding and working the twelve-step program. Thank you so much!

Rev. Dr. Kev.

www.ingramcontent.com/pod-product-compliance
Lightning Source LLC
Chambersburg PA
CBHW060813270326
41929CB00002B/27